SUPERPOWERS ACTIVATE

A Guide to Empower Your Inner Superhero

TAMMY HOLT

Superpowers Activate/Tammy Holt

Paperback ISBN 978-1-7362177-0-2
Hardcover ISBN: 978-1-7362177-1-9
eBook ISBN: 978-1-7362177-2-6

DEDICATION

To God, you are mine; and I am yours forever. I am in you, you are in me, and there is only one of us.

To the fighter, rest, war, repeat.

To the dreamer, never stop...

CONTENTS

"Behold, I give unto you power to tread on serpents and scorpions, and over all the power of the enemy: and nothing shall by any means hurt you."

Luke 10:19

FOREWORD

What happens to a dream deferred?

Does it dry up

like a raisin in the sun?

Or fester like a sore—

And then run?

Does it stink like rotten meat?

Or crust and sugar over—

like a syrupy sweet?

Maybe it just sags

like a heavy load.

Or does it explode?

"*Harlem*" by Langston Hughes, 1951

MY SUPERPOWER STORY

I was born in the 70's on a military base. I am a motley mix of flower child, revolutionary, and dreamer. Like so many with a destiny greater than themselves, my story was in the making before I was born. It was coded in my DNA, like the monarch butterfly. They travel from Canada to Mexico, having never made the trek before. But the directions of their journey are written on their genes, passed down in their lineage as genetic memory. I find it amazing that the monarch knows where to go, and how to get there, while never having made the trip before. Like them, I am compelled to find a way, seek out truth, be a lioness for justice, and a lamb for peace.

I am the sum of many parts. The daughter of a child abandoned and rescued from a German orphanage in the 50's, who endured racism, domestic violence, and being a single-parent. She was the baby and woman that could not be broken. I am her seed that said, "I will repair the breach and find what was lost!" I am my grandmother's child. I thank her for thwarting the course of ill intent that was bent on dimming my destiny. Thank you for plucking my momma out of a room full of other "brown babies" unfairly forgotten and left to time. Granny's memory will forever be etched in my heart. Her redeeming, charismatic, warrior, and Queen Mother spirit lives on in me. May she rest in power!

I was created out of that mixture of fire and ice; high waters, winds, storms, and rust; barren, with dry bones, and beautifully broken; but still I stand. When I think of my life's journey, I am certain to have confused them all. I'm sure the fire inquires, "Why is that we burn her, yet she is not consumed?" The waters, perplexed, ask, "How is it that we rise, yet she walks on us?" The winds chime in, confused, "Who is she, that she makes even us calm?"

In May of 1997, I accepted Jesus Christ as my personal savior. My life has never been the same. There have been ups, downs, turns, and plot twists. But I've had Jesus as the captain of my ship, putting out fires, calming the winds, navigating the seas, and quieting the storms. There is a quote that sums it up nicely, "Fate whispers to the warrior, 'You cannot withstand the storm.' 'The warrior whispers back, 'I am the storm.'"[1] It is through Jesus' power that I am bold enough to talk back to the storm. It is rendered powerless. Jesus is my reckoning force; the reason I still stand.

I wage war against the dark forces. I charge my brothers and sisters in Christ to stand firm and rooted in the word of God. We are the true champions: victorious, reigning queens and kings; a royal priesthood with crowns on our heads. I look forward to the day when we can cast our crowns before God. We will never be defeated. My hope is that you find your fighting spirit and acknowledge your superpowers. Wear your superhero cape when you need an extra push to feel your greatness. May God's peace and power be with you. Superpowers Activate!

Your Superpower Ambassador,

Tammy Holt

"Let there be love, but if there has to be war: Let Us Fight!"

WHY I WROTE THIS BOOK

Have you ever wished you could fly, bend bars of steel, or lift a car with mental or physical strength? I have, and my coveted superpower of all is the ability to defy time and space. Oh, what fun would it be to time travel? The idea of traveling to the future (or past) to save the present (or future) is mind-boggling. Over 2000 years ago, that's exactly what Jesus did. His accomplishment on the cross set the future on an incredible course. He is the ultimate time traveler! What He did in the past rendered all of our sins (present, past, and future) powerless.

This book may not actually teach you to bend steel or time travel. But it will help lead the way to the incredible feats you will do. Using the authority of Jesus, our saving Christ, you can do all things! [2,3]

In the year of the 2020 pandemic, before the quarantine shut down, I went on a humanitarian trip to Peru with my church. While I thought my mission was to complete the tasks at-hand, and humbly serve the Peruvian people, God had other plans for me. It was there that I received overwhelming love and a Superhero's Cape! That cape gave me the confidence to write the book God has been prodding me to write for years.

My assignment was clear. Everywhere I looked, I saw the superpower theme. God's gentle nudging reminded me on several occasions to, "Just write the book, already!" I feel my mission in life is to repair the breach in hearts and mindsets. I was born to write this book for you and for me. I came to the realization that the book didn't have to be a dissertation or a thousand pages, only a few points to provide encouraging words to help someone experiencing life's challenges. I hope it will be a resource to help war against the darkness—and win!

If you want to experience the superpower mentioned in this book, ask Jesus to come into your life right now. Confess your sins and ask for forgiveness. Believe that He died for you and that you want Him to be your Lord and Savior.[4] You will have a never-ending relationship with a best friend, a superhero, a king! You will become a royal heir in a family of believers and receive the gifts and promises of God.

HOW TO USE THIS BOOK

Superpowers Activate is a guide to empower your inner superhero. It is a superpower manual of sorts: part inspirational and part workbook. It contains biblical scriptures directing and referring the reader back to the source of all greatness. God is the source of all things, including the "power" in our "Superpower." This book was created as a reminder that superpowers come from God's unrelenting grace and enduring love. These superpowers are our birthright as Christians.

Our superpower origin is detailed in the scriptures. After the war in Heaven, the enemy was cast out. Jesus was born with an important mission. His death, burial, and resurrection resulted in the gift of everlasting life; and a life filled with richness and abundancy. Isn't that exciting news? In addition to receiving everlasting life, He wanted us to also have abundant life while on earth. It is important to understand this *abundancy* concept. It means *"present in great quantity; more than adequate; over-sufficient; plentiful, rich, lavish, existing or available in large quantiles."*[5] Jesus wants us to have that kind of life! It is fundamental and the foundation of this book. It is Jesus' death that gave us power and authority. He is the ruler of all.[6]

After accepting Jesus as our personal savior, His power transferred to us. Jesus said, "Most assuredly, I say to you, he who believes in Me, the works that I do he will do also; and greater works than these he will do."[7] That sounds like superpower talk to me! It is this Christian faith that keeps me going when I want to quit.

The goal of this book is to help you engage and activate your superpowers for good. It is a guide to help bring out your super-hero qualities and warrior strength mentality. Pray and ask God to help you understand the scriptures, study and meditate on them daily; and they will empower you. Refer to the endnote scrip-tures, use the Superpower Workbook, and journal your thoughts, ideas, notes, and artwork in the blank space provided.

DISCLAIMER

Why superpowers? I can hear someone, somewhere, saying, "Why do we need to focus on having superpowers, or being a superhero? And not all superheroes wear capes." I hear you. But the point of this book is to inspire, encourage, and empower. To bring out the inhibited little girl or little boy, man or woman, to inspire them to dream unabated; to ignite their power; and the passion they already possess. My prayer and hope is that you dream freely (wear your cape and activate your superpowers)!

Also, I want to talk about the idea of PERFECTION. No one is perfect. The Bible says, "There is none righteous, no, not one."[8] This means NO ONE: not pastors, presidents, parents, friends, you, or me. We are imperfect. But through Jesus, His death makes us perfect in his eyes. If we have a repentant heart; and confess our sins to him, He will forgive us.[9] How Jesus makes my imperfection perfection is His inner mystery.

Although I strive for perfection in everything I do, this book is not perfect. I'm probably one of the least qualified to write it. God loves to show his strength in the meek, humble, and weak. I am certain He will make this imperfect book perfect for the one who needs it. This was my assignment from God. My "paralysis of over-analysis" is over. I've given it my best shot. Please take whatever mistakes or omissions you find with love.

The views and opinions in this book are mine. Read the Bible for yourself and ask God to reveal His truth to you.

WHAT IS A SUPERPOWER?

"A superpower is a power or ability (such as the ability to become invisible or to fly) of the kind possessed by superheroes: a superhuman power"[10]

Superpower Charge: Activate Your Superpowers!

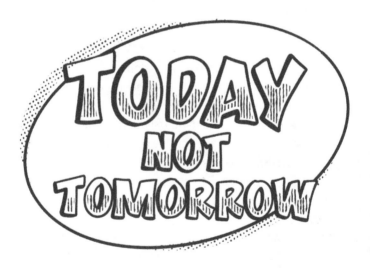

Where do you think superpower stories began? I like to think that the superhero characters originated as a way to explain the extraordinary. Superhero "...stories inspire us and provide models of coping with adversity, finding meaning in loss and trauma, discovering our strengths and using them for a good purpose."[11]

When I think of superpowers, the Hulk, Superman, Black Panther, and Wonder Woman come to mind. The world is infatuated with superheroes and superpowers. We watch as they are portrayed on TV and film, with endless sequels and die-hard cult followings. You can find their images on everything from t-shirts, pens, hats, and mugs.

There is this unusual connection between fantasy and science, where the fantastic wittily, and surprisingly, evade the scientific. And, if there is a hero, not too far away, you will find an antithesis, an archetype—a villain. Co-existing, there is this constant battle where evil tries to overcome good. The interesting thing about good and light is that if there is the tiniest sparkle, one drop, it invades the darkness. The Bible says that darkness does not comprehend light.

> *"In the beginning was the Word, and the Word was with God, and the Word was God. He was in the beginning with God. All things were made through Him, and without Him nothing was made that was made. In Him was life, and the life was the light of men. And the light shines in the darkness, and the darkness did not comprehend it."*[12]

According to this verse, because everything was made through Jesus, humans have His light. This shining light (that shines even in darkness) is what makes evil so mad. It's as if the evil in the world illuminates good all the more! Whatever the plight or circumstances we experience here on earth, Heaven, and God's host of angels are always rooting for us to win.[13]

The Word of God is living and breathing; it is a constant light to the world.[14] It is powerful and dynamic. The word dynamite actually comes from the Greek word *Dunamis* which means power. In the Bible, this word is used to describe God's word as explosive.

Let us be light. Walk in authority and power. Walk in the super-power, beaming, explosive light!

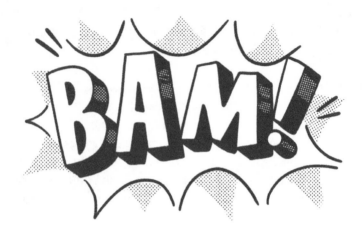

THE CHRISTIAN'S SUPERPOWERS

"I will praise You, for I am fearfully and wonderfully made; marvelous are Your works, and that my soul knows very well."[15]

"You are gods, and all of you are children of the Most High."[16]

Superpower Charge: You are Powerful! Walk in Authority!

The first dream I recall as a child, I was fighting evil. I was about 5 or 6 years old but can still vividly remember the dream. The scene was set during ancient or medieval times. I was dressed in a soldier's uniform, and was fighting in hand-to-hand combat. I remember all of these details. It is beyond my explanation to remember this as a child, but I do.

In the dream, God told me that you cannot fight evil with your hands. God said, "I have to fight your battles, and it occurs in the spiritual realm." I was too young to really know what it all meant. But I knew I wanted to learn to fight like that. It took many lessons and years of experience before I learned how, and I am still learning. I am a work in progress.

The Bible tells us that before we are born, God knows everything about us. He uniquely designed each one of us with detailed specifications. [17] He even knows the number of hairs on our head, and when we cry, captures our tears in a bottle. [18] Fearfully and wonderfully made, unfortunately, we often lack the confidence to walk in our God-given right, authority, and power (i.e., superpower).

I parallel our Christian powers to that of the superheroes in the movies. From the mere ordinary, we watch and admire as they morph into a totally different creature (with their capes and special powers) activated to do good and carry out the superhero creed, "Serve and Protect." Most superheroes' family and friends don't recognize them when they have on their capes. Alchemy happens, and their strength becomes unmatched, unrecognizable. They go by day-to-day looking like ordinary people, but they possess extraordinary prowess.

Similarly, when we accepted Jesus Christ as our personal savior. There was a rebirth, alchemy at its finest. We became new creations in Christ. [19] Born again, just like the superheroes who experience their transformation from some odd event. We are, by our very Christian nature, a superpower creation. God created us with His own mighty hand! Likewise, He gave us dominion over all creation. [20] It still amazes me how we can domesticate wild animals and create anything we put our hands to do.

As these superpowers may be unbelievable to others, they may even be elusive to you. Some did not believe Jesus was God in human form, here to save the world. So, just know people may not understand your so-called gift or superpower. That's okay. It's not about them. It's about you. Work on crafting and developing yourself to show yourself approved.[21] Continue to study and ask God for wisdom and strength in areas in which you are weak. Step into your superpower rite of passage.

You may not always feel very superpower-ish. And that's okay, too. Hold tight to your faith, ride the storm out. It is only a season; and it too, shall pass.[22]

SUPERPOWER STRATEGIES, TOOLS, AND WEAPONS

THE CAPE

"Bring the cloak that I left with Carpus at Troas when you come—and the books, especially the parchments."[23]

Superpower Charge: Where's My Cape?!

In this scripture, Paul was asking for his cloak to be brought to him. Can you just anticipate where I'm going with this?! Was this his superpower cloak (a.k.a. cape)? I know I'm stretching it a bit here, but it sure does make for good storytelling, lore, and imagination. Why was the cloak so important to mention in scripture? Why did he need it? I guess we will never know. But there is something special about cloaks and coats in the Bible. Not only do they provide warmth (which is the obvious); they specifically convey and indicate status. Similar to today, we know when someone has on a nice coat! Even Joseph received a special coat of many colors from his father, Jacob. It expressed his father's favor and that he would one day assume leadership over the family. His brothers did not like that; and envied him and his coat.

We will explore the "parchments" (i.e., books) more in the upcoming section.

23

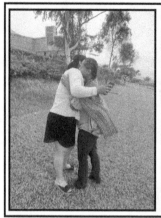
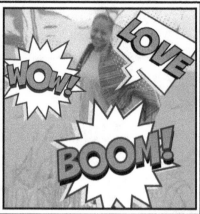

My Cape Story

I want to share with you my personal cape story. This is a Peruvian shawl that I received on the last day of the missionary trip. It is from a beautifully spirited and precious woman in Peru. It is my first Superhero Cape.

I wasn't expecting it and was overwhelmed with emotion. I was caught off guard, so there wasn't enough time to form a wall of strength and pride. I cried right there, just like a baby. It felt as if God himself was giving me a coat of many colors.

The cape is an illustration. It shows what happens in the spiritual realm, that I have a divine authority and covering. I didn't understand what God was telling me in Peru. Not until months later did I grasp the Holy Spirit's nudge: "I want you to walk in power, like a real super being with supernatural power, the power that God gave you."

What if the cape could give me special powers? What if, it alone, would help me to love the mean-spirited and "hard-lovables;"

to forgive the brute and the beast; to conjure up just enough gospel love dust to blow into their eyes (that would compel them to become 'a kind human')? For the record, it didn't. Although beautiful, it wasn't magical. I'm working on myself every day and asking God to give me this supernatural power.

The cape does, however, serve as a gentle reminder that I am powerful beyond measure. It signifies that I have a supernatural cape wrapped around me in the heavenly realm that is able to bring down strongholds and weapons (through prayers and fasting). It reminds me that all things are possible, and that NOTHING will be impossible to me, because I love God.

When we accepted Jesus as our personal savior, there was a change. We were born again and transformed. We became new creations in Christ! We walk, now, not in our own authority; but in His!

I think we can all agree that life is tough. There is no sugar-coating it. Either we are fighting our own negative thoughts or fending off the negative comments of others. We need as many tools in the toolbox to make it through one day to the next. A cape helps me tap into my inner superhero character in preparation for whatever the day brings. It represents the power that I already have in Jesus.

I think of how Joseph must have felt, honored and noble, with this coat of many colors. But how his brothers envied him. I'm sure there will be someone hating, saying, "Who do you think you are with that cape?" Don't let that discourage you! Step into your greatness and don your superpowers and cape for the world to see.

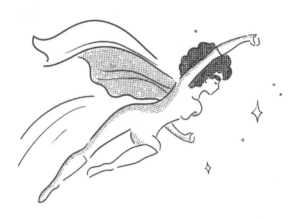

ASSIGNMENT:

This is the point in the book where you put on your cape. Do it today! Buy one or create it out of a bed sheet or towel. Wear it proudly and envision your superpowers activating! I'd love to hear all about it, email me with a picture and personal story.

THE BOOKS

"This Book of the Law shall not depart from your mouth, but you shall meditate in it day and night, that you may observe to do according to all that is written in it. For then you will make your way prosperous, and then you will have good success."[24]

Superpower Charge: Superpowers Activate: Charge and Recharge!

Our authority is the Holy Bible, which includes the Old and New Testament. Sixty-six books to be exact. One day, I saw a lady with a sweatshirt that said, "Genesis to Revelation, I Believe it All." That pretty much sums it up! I believe it all. It is our daily bread.

Daily meditation and devotion on God's word are necessary to set the tone of the day. His word activates superpowers, even when you're not aware of it happening. For example, you don't know how much you know or don't know in the class, until you take the test. The word of God has power, and as the Creator, He creates power in us. Studying His word helps prepare us for life's daily trials, tests, and challenges. When the fiery arrows of evil come, the word of God will have prepared you to endure. Your faith will render the fire or the storm powerless.

Paul mentioned that he needed his "parchments" for a reason. This subtle and short scripture has my imagination running wild. Superhero books and capes—oh my!! The word of God was the source of his strength. I'm sure those parchments had some exciting and encouraging information. There were so many things written about Jesus (back then and now). The world cannot contain them all.[25]

But what did those parchments say? The curiosity is killing me!

Aside from the fun and mystery of theorizing about Paul's parchments, set time aside to read the Bible. Also, find a devotional book that you can follow each day. There are different themes, lengths, and sizes to suit an individual's style. Establish a regular time and location to commune with God; when you rise in the morning and before you go to bed. It might be difficult to do with all of life's competing factors. But the goal is to have a conversation with the Creator of the Day, to find out how you should create yours. In the stillness, He will help settle you with His peace that surpasses all understanding.[26] Devotional time will get you ready for whatever crazy the day brings.

I've included a few resources in the back of the book to help jumpstart your research.

THE FUEL

Superpower Charge: Take Care of Your Temple!

The Bible story about Daniel provides some solid instructions on healthy living and eating. Daniel, Hananiah, Mishael, and Azariah (a.k.a. Belteshazzar, Meshach, Shadrach, and Abednego) stood firm against King Nebuchadnezzar's orders, and chose not to defile their bodies with the king's food. Instead, they consumed vegetables and water for 10 days. They proved to be in better condition than the king's soldiers.[27]

There are different types of spiritual fasts to include, but not limited to the Daniel Fast; an absolute water fast; not eating or drinking at all; or abstaining from social media. Whichever you choose, it's between you and God. The common denominator is praying and reading your scriptures. Remember, a superhero's fuel source is from God, and fasting is a crucial element of the Christian lifestyle.[28]

THE BRAVE, THE BOLD, AND THE FEARLESS

"For God has not given us a spirit of fear, but of power and of love and of a sound mind."[29]

"So he answered, 'Do not fear, for those who are with us are more than those who are with them.'"[30]

"Be strong and of good courage, do not fear nor be afraid of them; for the Lord your God, He is the One who goes with you. He will not leave you nor forsake you."[31]

Superpower Charge: Be Brave!

Being brave does not mean that the spirit of fear doesn't come knocking. It means you don't let it in to call the shots. Capture, neutralize, and subjugate these negative thoughts and arrows. Align them next to what the word of God says.

For example, if the voice says, "I'm scared," speak the word of God back to it: *"The Lord is my light and salvation; Whom Shall I Fear?"*[32] This will help render the negative thinking powerless. Remember, only light can cast out darkness. Be persistent as you recite scripture back to yourself.

With these principles in mind, do whatever God has called you to do with **BOLDNESS**. God did not give us a spirit of fear. So being brave means to exhibit courage while still facing the threat.[33]

One great example of bravery and boldness occurred during David's youth. The Bible says he was young, yet fearless. This dude was so bad that he wasn't afraid of giants or lions. One of my favorite quotes was said by David regarding Goliath. I say it when

I am encountering fear, *"Who is this uncircumcised Philistine that he should defy the armies of the living God?"*[34] I'm one of those soldiers in the Army of the Living God! So that devil, (or mean person at work, that spirit of depression, whatever it is) has to back up off me! God's got my back! I ask God, my *Abba* (Father) to fight on my behalf! Focus on your faith in God rather than fear. Speak life and positivity over yourself, and remember to pray to God for strength and reinforcement.

So, whatever you encounter in life, look it square in the eyes (in a spiritual or physical sense) with God towering over your back in protection mode while you fight. In other biblical stories, God went before His people to slay the enemies (so that they didn't even have to fight). Our God is amazing, and it's comforting to know that the battle is not ours but His.[35]

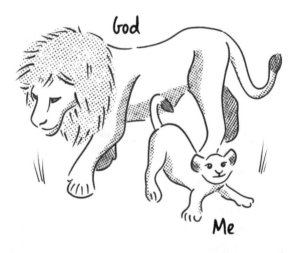

What makes David's story more incredible is that God gave David the ability to slay Goliath with one single, smooth stone. He cracked this giant's head wide open. BAM!! Then, he cut his head off as a token of triumph. I love that part. The towering, huge, literal giant, that everyone else was afraid of, was killed with a rock! The shepherd boy did what the well-trained soldiers could not. So, the point is, don't focus on your own ability, but remember the battle belongs to God. Your superpower could be as small as a rock, but mighty!

There are other stories in the Bible where additional attempts had to be made to reach the victory. Some cases will require more than one try. Don't get discouraged on your first, second, or seventh attempt. For example, it took marching around Jericho's walls 7 times before they fell. In these cases, when your hope gets challenged, know that God is always in control. If you are aligned with Christ, and it's in His will, it will come to pass. Patience may be the test. In other cases, it may not be God's will. Pray for understanding and peace, so that God will settle your heart on the matter.

Another favorite scripture is when God held time up.[36] Yes, time actually stood still to give God's people an advantage in battle. Our God is the Father of Time. This was an easy task for God, but an amazing and awesome event for Joshua to experience during battle.

You talk about some inspiring examples on how to be—

Bold!

Brave!

Fearless!

I know it's not always easy, and you'll have to train like the superheroes do to keep your warrior fighter skills intact. Reading the word of God every day will give you the training and strength you need. Think of it as a daily bread to create brave, bold, and fearless muscles. Meditate on His word day and night. Contemplate it, ponder it, and ask God to clarify things that are ambiguous.

Try to memorize the scriptures that speak to you and your situation. My go-to scriptures that help me deal with fear and inadequacy are *Psalm 27* and *Psalm 23*. Even if you can only retain a handful of verses, they will help you when needed.

When you feel fear creeping in, think of what Jesus did when He died on the cross for our sins. He did what no other person could do (no one, ever). He got out of the grave with all power. The scriptures tell us that He went into the very gates of Hades and set the captives free.[37] That's a quintessential superpower if you ask me. His death gave us the right to boldly and freely come to Him. We don't need a priest, pastor, or anyone to talk to God for us. Jesus tore the veil that allows us heavenly access at all times.[38] God loves us so much that He gave us His only begotten son that we should not perish, but have everlasting life AND have power while on earth.

Blessed be your coming in and going out, SUPERHEROES!

Know this, as believers in Jesus, we have power over air, water, and fire! Jesus commanded the wind, He walked on water, and came into the burning fire with Daniel (and was not consumed)![39] Therefore, "Do not be afraid," we have the same powers to slay giants with one stone and withstand fire. Jesus will be in the fire with us; and the storm will not overtake us; you can command the seas; the winds will even bow down to us; let's walk on this water together! With Jesus, all things are possible!

Say it again! Let me hear a bold and brave war cry! Say a *HALLE-LUJAH*, it is a praise that will confuse the enemy!!

The scripture's caution that you be doers of the word, and not hearers only. For if anyone is a hearer of the word and not a doer, he is like a man who looks in a mirror and forgets his own face.[40] Don't be like that person. Always remember your inner superhero.

THE PRAYER POWER

"Be anxious for nothing, but in everything by prayer and supplication, with thanksgiving, let your request be made known to God."[41]

Superpower Charge: Go Pray!

Prayer is the tool to access your divine superpower. It is during prayer that we communicate with God.

Prayer does not involve magical words or creative repetitions.[42] The best model is the Lord's Prayer. The commonly known acronym A.C.T.S can help.[43]

A for Adoration—praising and honoring God
C for Confession—confessing your sins to God
T for Thanksgiving—telling God you are thankful for all that He has done for you
S for Supplication—pray that God supplies your needs and the needs of others

Prayer Powers fire up!

LET'S GO!

THE LOVE POWER

*"Darkness cannot drive out darkness: only light can do that. Hate
cannot drive out hate: only love can do that."*
Martin Luther King Jr.

Superpower Charge: Love the Hell Out of Them!

Love is the greatest superpower of all.[44] If we love hard enough,
we can love the HELL right out of anyone or any situation. Love
will extinguish fire and melt away any wretched ice that exists.
I know it sounds cliché and easy to do. But in reality, it isn't.
It takes real superpower to love the mean-spirited, the hate-
ful, unjust, and the bitterly wounded. Especially when there are
parts within our own selves that feel the same spirits of hurt,
bitterness, brokenness, or betrayal. It might take time and require patience; but with prayer, something in the supernatural
realm will break. The Love Power can break down the tallest and
toughest walls.

Remember: A superhero's number one weapon is love. Love is
infectious. "Greater love has no one other than this, than to lay
down one's life for his friends."[45]

The superhero path is not easy. It requires discipline and humil-
ity.[46] God loves the humble. I've had to love people that laughed
at me and said mean things to me. But God said, don't take
everything to heart.[47] He also said that a fool says everything on
his mind.[48] Say less, love more. Reflect on these tenets as you go
about your superhero day.

Although I've dealt with betrayal and friendships lost, God keeps
on blessing me and raising me up above my enemies. He will do

that for you, too. Most of all, I have a forever-friend in Jesus. His love has kept me going and helps me to love the next person harder than the last.

I hope this book will empower you to love the "hard-loveables," too. And it's okay to love some people from afar. Someone causing you mental or physical harm should not be brought (or kept) into your life. Pray for them, and love them in your heart (but again, from afar).

My superpower charge: let us be Christ imitators! His way of compassion, forgiveness, self-denial, and love. He said to love your neighbor as yourself.[49] We don't have to always agree with our neighbor to love them. Love what God loves; abhor what He hates. Following God's commandments may not always be popular among men. But do what is pleasing to God; and be popular in His eyes. We are the light among the darkness. Walk boldly as the light!

And, last, but definitely not least. L.O.V.E., L.O.V.E., L.O.V.E., yourself! Wrap your arms around the only person whose skin you are in, and give yourself a big hug!

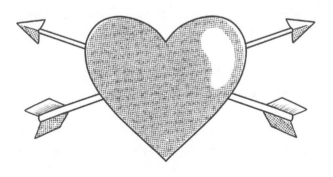

THE WAY WE WAR

"Finally, my brethren, be strong in the Lord and in the power of His might. Put on the whole armor of God, that you may be able to stand against the wiles of the devil. For we do not wrestle against flesh and blood, but against principalities, against powers, against the rulers of the darkness of this age, against spiritual hosts of wickedness in the heavenly places. Therefore take up the whole armor of God, that you may be able to withstand in the evil day, and having done all, to stand. Stand therefore, having girded your waist with truth, having put on the breastplate of righteousness, and having shod your feet with the preparation of the gospel of peace; above all, taking the shield of faith with which you will be able to quench all the fiery darts of the wicked one. And take the helmet of salvation, and the sword of the Spirit, which is the word of God; praying always with all prayer and supplication in the Spirit, being watchful to this end with all perseverance and supplication for all the saints..."[50]

"For though we walk in the flesh, we do not war according to the flesh. For the weapons of our warfare are not carnal but mighty in God for pulling down strongholds, casting down arguments and every high thing that exalts itself against the knowledge of God, bringing every thought into captivity to the obedience of Christ..."[51]

Superpower Charge: The Battle is Not Yours, It's God's!

As superheroes for Christ, we fight not with our hands, but with all the tools and strategies God has given us. We have the scriptures, prayer and fasting, and an empowered mindset to include being brave, bold, and fearless. We know that love always wins, and light always illuminates the darkness.

In Biblical times, God's people had to fight in actual wars. Although we remember those stories of how God trained His peoples' hands for war, we let God fight our battles in the spiritual realm.[52] Do not war according to the flesh, but put on the whole armor of God, as mentioned in Ephesians 6.

Don't let negative voices use kryptonite (i.e., the only stone that can make Superman defenseless) to pierce through your powers, your posture, strides, or empowered mind. The voices will come and go. Just know that every thought you should examine. Every thought is not always yours; some are implanted or staged at just the right time to make you think it came from within, when in actuality it's evil, negative, demonically orchestrated; implanted by the enemy. Lies spoken over you or told to you even by trusted people cannot maintain residence in the superhero's mind. They have got to go!

Identify your kryptonite and ways to respond when you encounter it. Don't let that thing that's hurtful, painful, and even unexpected <u>from</u> someone unexpected rule your life. If you live long enough (as my Granny would say), you will experience some sort of a trial, test, or tribulation. Be not discouraged. Jesus tells us that he overcame the world and for us to be of good cheer.[53]

Wait, what did that say?

Be of good cheer? How can we be cheerful during an unhappy situation? Simply, BE HAPPY in spite of and through it all. Smile when you want to frown. Laugh when you want to cry. Pray for and bless the person you really want to curse out! It all sounds counter-intuitive (especially, when you are hurting or in pain yourself); but only light can cast out darkness. Joy can only cast out sadness. This attitude will render the kryptonite and fiery darts powerless. This is an example of the superpower mindset.

Rest, War, and Repeat. This is the way we war!

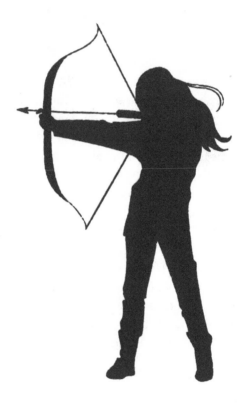

THE INNER SUPERHERO

"I will send out an army to find you, In the middle of the darkest night. It's true, I will rescue you, I will never stop marchin' to reach you, In the middle of the hardest fight, it's true, I will rescue you..."[54]

Superpower Charge: Leave the 99!

In these lyrics, Lauren Daigle, sings about God coming to rescue us, and how He will never stop trying to reach us. Jesus wants us all to receive the gift of salvation, so our goal is to always be on the lookout for the one that needs our help. That's what Superheroes do. Scan the room, be ready for the prodding of the Holy Spirit to tell you who to help (even if it's just a kind word or praying for them).

There is a scripture that talks about leaving the 99 for one. There might be 100 sheep, but if one goes missing, the shepherd goes looking to bring it home. Jesus is like that with us. He is the Good Shepherd. We can apply it to modern-day times by saying, we should leave the comfort of ourselves, our shells (if you are an introverted extrovert, like me), and our homes to find the one that needs encouragement or salvation. Just as someone came for us, we have to pay it forward and find the next one to help. One of our great superhero abilities is to go after the missing one.[55]

It is also a Christian's great commission to spread the gospel to all nations.[56] Let's make Jesus proud!

Now, go forth and multiply!

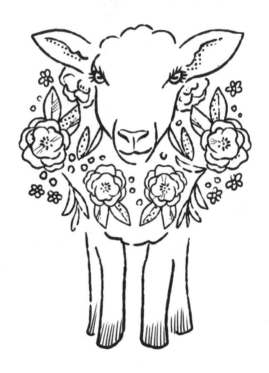

THE REAL SUPERMAN

"Therefore God also has highly exalted Him and given Him the name which is above every name, that at the name of Jesus every knee should bow, of those in heaven, and of those on earth, and of those under the earth, and that every tongue should confess that Jesus Christ is Lord, to the glory of God the Father."[57]

"Let this mind be in you which was also in Christ Jesus, who, being in the form of God, did not consider it robbery to be equal with God, but made Himself of no reputation, taking the form of a bond-servant, and coming in the likeness of men. And being found in appearance as a man, He humbled Himself and became obedient to the point of death, even the death of the cross."[58]

Superpower Charge: Charge, Recharge, and Charge Again!

The real superman is Jesus. He is God. He came down in human form to set the captives free. He sits in Heaven on the throne and helps us to fight our daily battles. He is our real-life superhero. Let us imitate Him! We should be on a perpetual recharge by staying in His presence through studying, praying, and fasting. REPEAT!

Brothers and sisters in Christ, put on your cape and full armor of God. Identify your superpower and use it. Ask God to reveal it to you. We are more than conquerors in Christ Jesus. Submit your life to Him, and He will do more than you can ever think or ask. The world needs us to step into our destiny. We serve a real Superman. There is none like Him. As His children, we have access to those same superpowers. He said that you will do even greater miracles than His. Read that again! Greater miracles than Jesus?[59] Wow that's deep...take a moment and meditate on that.

Superpowers ACTIVATE!

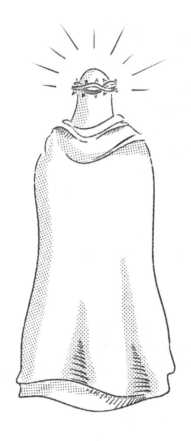

THE SUPERHERO WORKBOOK

This is the Superhero Workbook. Review the next sections with an empowered mindset. The first section is the Superpower Assessment. The following sections cover the Christian Fighter, the War, the Opponent, and the Victory. Use the blank space to fill in your answers. You can also access a free Superhero Discussion Guide for scriptures on spiritual warfare at www.superpowers-activate.org.

THE
SUPERPOWER
ASSESSMENT

What are your superpowers?

_____

_____

_____

_____

_____

_____

If you are having trouble identifying your superpowers, list things that you are passionate about, good at doing, or want to learn to do.

_____

_____

_____

_____

_____

_____

_____

How can you use your gifts (i.e. superpowers) to glorify God and His kingdom?

_____

_____

_____

_____

_____

_____

_____

_____

_____

_____

_____

_____

_____

_____

THE
CHRISTIAN
FIGHTER

List examples of different types of fighters.

_____

_____

_____

_____

_____

_____

How does a Christian prepare for battle?

_____

_____

_____

_____

_____

_____

_____

_____

How do you overcome fear?

_____

_____

_____

_____

_____

_____

_____

_____

_____

_____

_____

_____

_____

_____

_____

_____

THE WAR

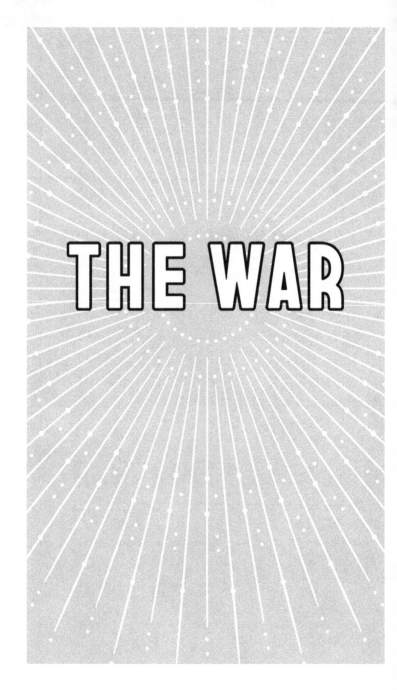

What is warfare?

_____

_____

_____

_____

Can you list examples of warfare (physical or mental)?

_____

_____

_____

_____

What does it mean to fight?

_____

_____

_____

_____

_____

_____

_____

Why do Christians have to fight?

_____

_____

_____

_____

_____

_____

How do Christians fight?

_____

_____

_____

_____

_____

_____

_____

THE
OPPONENT

What is an opponent?

_____

_____

_____

_____

_____

_____

_____

Who is our opponent?

_____

_____

_____

_____

_____

_____

_____

_____

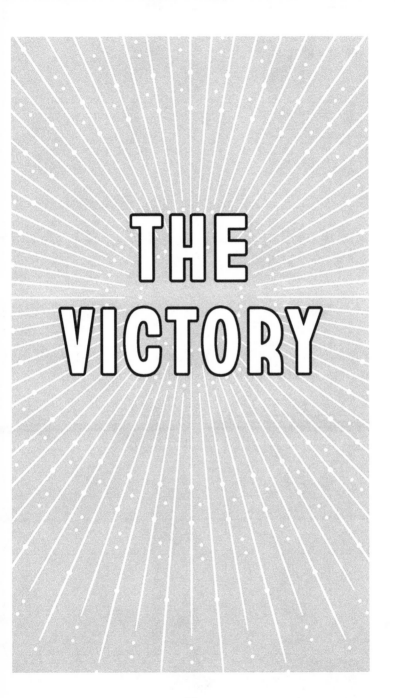

THE VICTORY

What is a victory?

_____

_____

_____

_____

_____

_____

_____

What gift has God given you to be victorious?

_____

_____

_____

_____

_____

_____

_____

_____

What is your Superpower Story?

_____

_____

_____

_____

_____

_____

_____

_____

_____

_____

_____

_____

_____

_____

_____

_____

RESOURCES

100 Days to Brave: Devotions for Unlocking Your Most Courageous Self by Annie F. Downs

Fasting for Breakthrough and Deliverance by John Eckhardt

Jesus Calling Morning and Evening Devotional by Sarah Young

Know What You Believe by Paul E. Little

Praying the Names of Jesus by Ann Spangler

Praying the Names of God by Ann Spangler

The 40-Day Surrender Fast by Celeste Camille Owens

The Battle is the Lord's by Tony Evans

The Resolution for Women by Priscilla Shirer

www.fbcglenarden.org

www.SuperpowersActivate.org

ACKNOWLEDGMENTS

I thank my precious husband, Patrick, for his unrelenting support in all that my hands have fashioned to do over the years. I tried to keep this book a surprise. But I know he found it strange all the capes, and superpower t-shirts laying around the house (or either tied around my neck). You are my king. You will always be my superhero. I adore you and your remarkable superpowers!

Every superhero has a crew of super friends and family; you know who you are. You are my life; you are my air. I especially thank my Momma for allowing me to occupy her body and for the safe journey to planet earth.

I am grateful to all the soldiers and veterans of the United States armed forces for their service. You are the epitome of bravery. "Greater love hath no man than this, that a man lay down his life for his friends." Thank you for your sacrifice.

I thank First Baptist Church of Glenarden for teaching, training, and loving me. I especially thank Senior Pastor John K. Jenkins, Sr. and First Lady Trina Jenkins (Grace Girls Rock!) for your leadership and wisdom. I appreciate all the bishops; visiting pastors; deacons and deaconesses; mothers of the church; missionary teams; the Puppet Ministry; and Sisters in Discipleship (mothers and sisters). Your teachings were not in vain and are at the heart of this book.

I also thank Grand Master Roberts of Kim Studio in Rockville, Maryland; Master Jason Hill; Mr. Peter Butler; and all the staff and students for their insight on how to build patience, training, and character. They taught me how to physically train the body; take punches to the mid-section (I had the best abs of my life back then); and blows to the legs. The premise was that the body would get stronger and stronger from each hit as it rebuilt itself. Albeit this was in a controlled dojo setting, under the scrutiny and watchful eye of the higher-ranked belts. The experience provided insight into training the mind and body for fighting. Although I earned a black belt, the white belt was the hardest. It required this then 30-year-old to take her first karate class. I not only had to begin; but commit to the process.

Thanks to the Tiny Book team. I could not have done this without you. When I wanted to give up, you encouraged me to refocus, and remember the purpose. I am forever grateful.

ENDNOTES

1   Author Unknown cited by Jake Remington.

2   All scriptures are from the New King James Version.

3   Philippians 4:13

4   Romans 10:10; Romans 10:13

5   Dictionary.com

6   Colossians 2:10

7   John 14:12

8   Romans 3:10

9   1 John 1:9

10   https://www.merriam-webster.com/dictionary/super-power (Retrieved 6/15/2020)

11   https://www.smithsonianmag.com/arts-culture/the-psychology-behind-superhero-origin-stories-4015776/ (Retrieved 10/22/20)

12   John 1:1-5

13   Hebrews 12:1

14   Romans 1:16; Acts 1:8

15   Psalm 139:14

16   Psalm 82:6

17   Psalm 139

18   Luke 12:7; Psalm 56:8

19   2 Corinthians 5:17

20   Genesis 1:26

21   2 Timothy 2:15

22   Ecclesiastes 3:1-8

23   2 Timothy 4:13

24   Joshua 1:8

25   John 21:25

26   Philippians 4:7

27   Daniel 1

28   Ezra 8:23; Matthew 17:21

29   2 Timothy 1:7

30   2 Kings 6:16

31   Deuteronomy 31:6

32   Psalm 27:1

33   Dictionary.com

34   1 Samuel 17:26

35   2 Chronicles 20

36   Joshua 10:13

37   Ephesians 4:9

38   Luke 23:45

39   Mark 4:35–41; Matthew 14:22–33; Daniel 3:25

40   James 1:22–25

41   Philippians 4:6

42   Matthew 6:7

43   Matthew 6:9–13

44   1 Corinthians 13:13

45   John 15:13

46   Psalm 138:6

47   Ecclesiastes 7:21

48   Proverbs 29:11

49   Matthew 19:19

50   Ephesians 6:10–18

51   2 Corinthians 10:3–6

52   Psalm 144

53   John 16:33

54   *Rescue* lyrics by Lauren Daigle

55   Mark 18:12

56   Matthew 28:19

57 Philippians 2:9–11
58 Philippians 2:5–8
59 John 14:12

CPSIA information can be obtained
at www.ICGtesting.com
Printed in the USA
LVHW031140250121
677402LV00006B/189

9 781736 217719